Using This Book

This page provides a brief guide to using this book.
Trail descriptions contain:

Trail Name

Trail Map with Roads and Contours

Red Lines Indicate Unpaved Trails

Solid Black Lines Indicate Paved Trails

Description of Trail Difficulty

Scenery Score

Detailed Trail Description

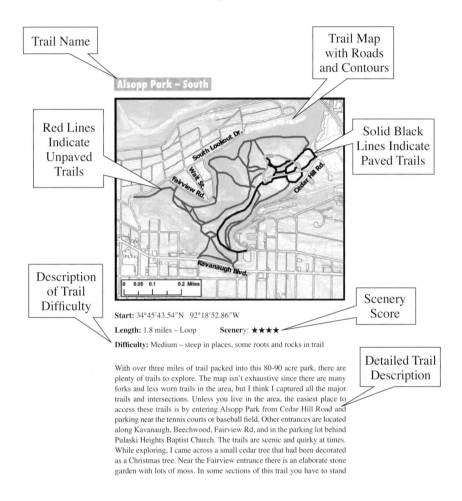

Alsopp Park – South

Start: 34°45′43.54″N 92°18′52.86″W

Length: 1.8 miles – Loop   **Scenery:** ★★★★

Difficulty: Medium – steep in places, some roots and rocks in trail

With over three miles of trail packed into this 80-90 acre park, there are plenty of trails to explore. The map isn't exhaustive since there are many forks and less worn trails in the area, but I think I captured all the major trails and intersections. Unless you live in the area, the easiest place to access these trails is by entering Alsopp Park from Cedar Hill Road and parking near the tennis courts or baseball field. Other entrances are located along Kavanaugh, Beechwood, Fairview Rd, and in the parking lot behind Pulaski Heights Baptist Church. The trails are scenic and quirky at times. While exploring, I came across a small cedar tree that had been decorated as a Christmas tree. Near the Fairview entrance there is an elaborate stone garden with lots of moss. In some sections of this trail you have to stand

GPS coordinates provided can be entered into Google Maps or Google Earth to help you get directions to each trailhead. ou can use a space instead of the degree symbol. For example, you would just type 34 50′22.26″N 92 29′34.64″W into the box on maps.google.com to find out where the West Summit Trailhead at Pinnacle is.

Many trailheads mentioned in this book are unmarked, so keep a careful eye out.

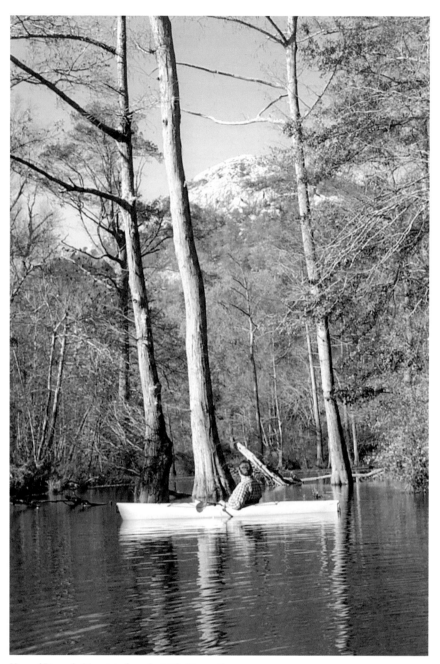

View of Pinnacle Mountain from the Little Maumelle.

TRAILS
OF LITTLE ROCK

A GUIDE TO LITTLE ROCK'S
LAND AND WATER TRAILS

HIKE • BIKE • PADDLE

Johnnie Chamberlin

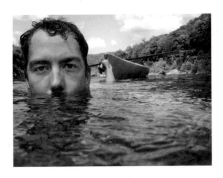

Parkhurst Brothers, Inc.
Little Rock, Arkansas

PREVIOUS PAGE: *The author enjoying Little Rock's water trails.*

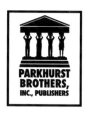

PARKHURST
BROTHERS,
INC., PUBLISHERS

www.pbros.net

Parkhurst Brothers books are distributed to the trade through the University of Chicago Press Distribution Center. Copies of this and other Parkhurst Brothers, Inc., Publishers titles are available to organizations and corporations for purchase in quantity by contacting Special Sales Department at our home office location, listed on our web site.

Printed in Canada

First Edition, 2009

12 11 10 9 8 7 6 5 4 3 2 1

Library of Congress LCCN: 2009922538

ISBN: 978-1-935166-10-8

This book is printed on archival-quality paper that meets requirements of the American National Standard for Information Sciences, Permanence of Paper, Printed Library Materials, ANSI Z39.48-1984.

Photographs used in this book are the property of the author or were secured for use in this book by the author. Used by permission of Little Rock Catholic High School, Little Rock, Arkansas.

Book design and cover design:	Wendell E. Hall
Page composition:	Shelly Culbertson
Acquired for Parkhurst Brothers, Inc., Publishers by:	Ted Parkhurst
Editor:	Rod Lorenzen
Project manager:	Ted Parkhurst

This book is dedicated
to Pops and Papaw.

Acknowledgments

This book never would have happened if it weren't for my dad and our use of his Tim Ernst books. He and his dad got me into hiking, backpacking, and boating. This book was also made possible by Audubon Arkansas which provided me with GIS training and the task of exploring lesser known areas of Little Rock.

Warning

Some of the trails in this book are in fairly isolated parts of the city. While I believe most of them are on public property, I'm not sure about all of them. Be sure to take adequate precautions and prepare for your trips! Many of the trips mentioned in here can take most of a day to complete, so be sure to take water and food on the longer ones.

Table of Contents

Introduction. 9
Trails Organized by Difficulty. 11
Trails by Region 12
Top 10's 13

Foot and Bike Trails. 15
  Alsopp Park 15
    Alsopp Park – North. 16
    Alsopp Park – South 17
  Boyle Park 19
  Boyle Park – East 20
    Southern Ridge Trail. 20
    Nun Trail. 22
    Archwood Winding Trail. 24
  Boyle Park – West. 26
    Boyle Park West Outer Trail 26
    Boyle Park West Inner Loop Trail 28
  Brodie Creek 29
    Upstream from Col. Glenn Rd. 30
    Between Brodie Creek Park and Hindman 32
  Gillam Park / Audubon Nature Center. 35
    Uplands Loop 36
    Bottomland Forest and Oxbow Loop 38
  Knoop Loop. 40
  Pinnacle Mountain 43
    East Summit 44
    West Summit 46
    Base Trail 48
    Kingfisher Trail 50
    Arboretum Trail 51
    Quarry Trail. 52
  River Mountain Park 54
  River Trail 56
    River Trail Loop from River Mountain Rd 56
  Rock Creek Trail 58
  Two Rivers Park 60
    Two Rivers Park – Paved Loop 61

Water Trails 63

   Fourche Creek 63

      Upper Section: I-430 – Benny Craig Park 62

      Middle Section: Benny Craig Park – Interstate Park 66

      Downstream Section: Interstate Park – Arkansas River 68

   Little Maumelle 71

      Little Maumelle: Pinnacle Mountain – Two Rivers Park 72

Potential/Upcoming Trails 75

   Coleman Creek Greenway Trail 76

   Rose Creek Trail 78

   Audubon Nature Center / Gillam Park 79

   Two Rivers Park 80

Introduction

I got the idea to write this book after working for Audubon Arkansas for two years. As part of my job I walked along all the major creeks in Little Rock and the surrounding areas. I also spent many days floating Fourche Creek searching for rare plants, planting trees, and clearing log jams. On the job, I came across several trails that I'd never heard about and most people I told about them had never heard of them either. What finally sealed the deal for me was when I moved to the Broodmoor neighborhood near Boyle Park. On my first few jogging excursions into that park I kept finding more and more trails that I never knew about. I thought if someone who enjoys our city parks and wild places as much as I do didn't know, then there must be lots of folks out there missing out on all the great places inside our city!

This book is not exhaustive, but contains information on dozens of great hikes, floats, and bike and pedestrian trails in the Little Rock area.

If you know of any trails I missed, feel free to e-mail me at johnnie.chamberlin@gmail.com and I will include it in any future editions of the book and credit you.

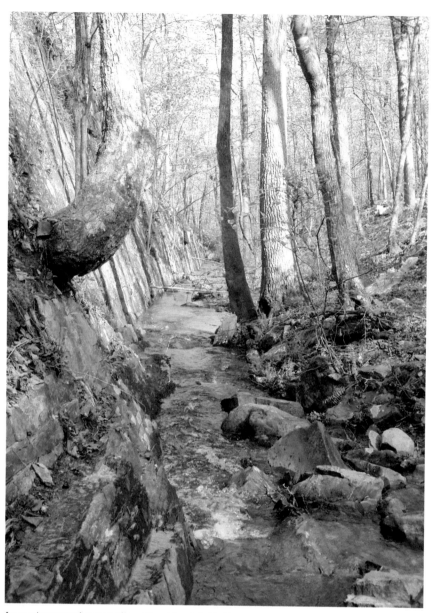

Interesting natural stone wall on River Mountain Trail.

Trails Organized by Difficulty

Easy

Water Trails. 63
Arboretum Trail – Pinnacle Mountain 51
Bottomland Forest and Oxbow Loop – Gillam Park 38
Brodie Creek Upstream from Col. Glenn Rd.. 30
Fourche Creek Lower Section. 68
Kingfisher Trail – Pinnacle Mountain 50
Knoop Loop – Knoop Park. 40
Paved Loop Trail – Two Rivers Park 61
River Trail. 56
Rock Creek Trail – Rock Creek Park. 58

Moderate

Alsopp Park North. 16
Alsopp Park South. 17
Base Trail – Pinnacle Mountain 48
Brodie Creek – Between Brodie Creek Park and Hindman 32
Fourche Creek – Upper Section 64
Little Maumelle River – Pinnacle Mountain to Two Rivers Park 72
Nun Trail – Boyle Park. 22
Quarry Trail – Pinnacle Mountain 52
River Mountain Park 54
Southern Ridge Trail – Boyle Park 20
Uplands Loop – Gillam Park. 36
West Inner Loop Trail – Boyle Park. 28
West Outer Trail – Boyle Park 26

Hard

East Summit – Pinnacle Mountain. 44
West Summit – Pinnacle Mountain 46
Archwood Windy Trail – Boyle Park. 24
Fourche Creek – Benny Craig to Interstate Park 66

Trails by Region

East Little Rock

Bottomland Forest and Oxbow Loop – Gillam Park 38
Fourche Creek Lower Section. 68
River Trail. 56
Uplands Loop – Gillam Park. 36

Central Little Rock

Alsopp Park North. 16
Alsopp Park South. 17
Archwood Windy Trail – Boyle Park. 24
Brodie Creek – Between Brodie Creek Park and Hindman 32
Fourche Creek Middle Section 66
Knoop Loop – Knoop Park. 40
Nun Trail – Boyle Park. 22
River Trail. 56
Southern Ridge Trail – Boyle Park 20
West Inner Loop Trail – Boyle Park. 28
West Outer Trail – Boyle Park 26

West Little Rock

Arboretum Trail – Pinnacle Mountain 51
Base Trail – Pinnacle Mountain 48
East Summit – Pinnacle Mountain. 44
West Summit – Pinnacle Mountain 46
Garden of Trees – Two Rivers Park 50
Little Maumelle River – Pinnacle Mountain to Two Rivers Park 72
Paved Loop Trail – Two Rivers Park 61
River Trail. 58
Rock Creek Trail – Rock Creek Park. 58
River Mountain Park 54
Quarry Trail – Pinnacle Mountain. 52

Southwest Little Rock

Brodie Creek Upstream from Col. Glenn Rd. 30
Fourche Creek Upper Section 64

Top 10's

Top 10 Most Scenic Trails:

1. Pinnacle Mountain East Summit Trail 44
2. River Trail 56
3. Pinnacle Mountain West Summit Trail 46
4. Little Maumelle 72
5. Fourche Creek Middle Section 66
6. Brodie Creek Upstream of Col. Glenn 30
7. Knoop Loop 40
8. Quarry Trail – Pinnacle Mountain 52
9. River Mountain Park 54
10. Paved Loop Trail – Two Rivers Park 61

Top 10 Trails for Kids:

1. River Trail 56
2. Paved Loop Trail – Two Rivers Park 61
3. Kingfisher Trail at Pinnacle Mountain 50
4. Boyle Park Bike/Pedestrian Trails 19
5. Pinnacle Mountain West Summit 46
6. Bottomland Forest and Oxbow Loop – Gillam Park 38
7. Alsopp Park South 17
8. Little Maumelle 72
9. Knoop Loop 40
10. Rock Creek Trail 58

Top 10 Trails for Solitude:

1. River Mountain Park 54
2. Brodie Creek Upstream of Col. Glenn 30
3. Fourche Creek Upper Section 64
4. Brodie Creek – Brodie Creek Park to Hindman 32
5. Fourche Creek Middle Section 66
6. Boyle Park West Outer Trail 26
7. Nun Trail 22
8. Archwood Windy Trail 24
9. Quarry Trail Pinnacle Mountain 52
10. Fourche Creek Lower Section 68

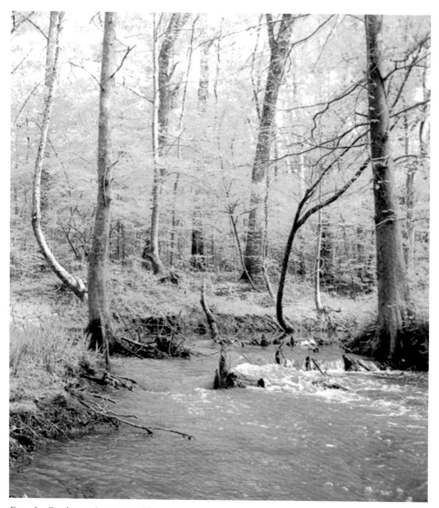

Fourche Creek near Interstate 430.

Foot and Bike Trails

ALSOPP PARK

Alsopp Park covers two valleys located between the Hillcrest and Riverdale neighborhoods of Little Rock. There are numerous dirt trails through the woods in this park as well as some improved/paved trails that are used by bikers as well as pedestrians.

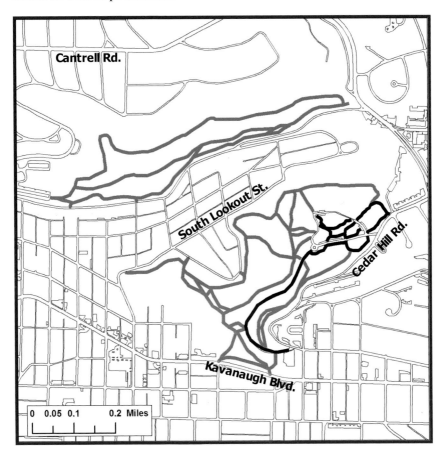

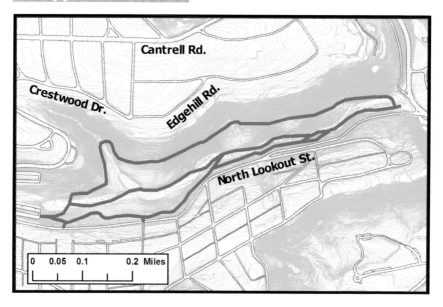

Start: 34°45′57.44″N   92°18′53.47″W

Length: 1.5 miles – Loop   **Scenery**: ★★★

Difficulty: Medium – Steep in places, some roots and rocks in trail

The main entrance to this trail is at the intersection of Cantrell and Alsopp Park Rd. There are more entrances along Lookout Rd and behind some apartments. This section of Alsopp consists of three trails that run roughly parallel to each other while following a creek channel. In general the most well worn trail is the middle trail, which follows a sewer right of way in several places. The most scenic trail is probably the northern route since it is the farthest from busy roads and the highest in elevation.

Park at the small parking lot at the main entrance. Hit the trail and stay right to get on the most scenic branch of the trail. The trail heads up rather steeply during the first 100 yards and then is fairly level for most of the next ¾ miles. The trail has a couple small bridges that cross streams that are small or dry except during and shortly after big rains when they turn into raging, breathtaking waterfalls. Where the trail forks, turn left and head back down the middle trail or stay right and explore the section of trail that runs along Lookout and eventually makes its way back down to the parking lot.

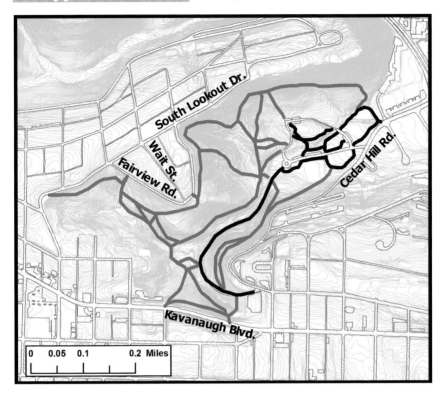

Start: 34°45'43.54"N   92°18'52.86"W

Length: 1.8 miles – Loop   **Scenery:** ★★★★

Difficulty: Medium – steep in places, some roots and rocks in trail

With over three miles of trail packed into this 80-90 acre park, there are plenty of trails to explore. The map isn't exhaustive since there are many forks and less worn trails in the area, but I think I captured all the major trails and intersections. Unless you live in the area, the easiest place to access these trails is by entering Alsopp Park from Cedar Hill Road and parking near the tennis courts or baseball field. Other entrances are located along Kavanaugh, Beechwood, Fairview Rd, and in the parking lot behind Pulaski Heights Baptist Church. The trails are scenic and quirky at times. While exploring, I came across a small cedar tree that had been decorated as a Christmas tree. Near the Fairview entrance there is an elaborate stone garden with lots of moss. In some sections of this trail you have to stand very still and listen quietly to realize you are in the city! The trails are easy to spot and pretty level and smooth most places, though there are some rocky and steep parts.

Starting at the parking lot near the tennis courts, head right on the paved trail next to the creek. After 100 yards, turn left onto the dirt trail and head up the hill. The trail is somewhat steep for the next 100 yards and then levels out. Stay right for the next ¾ mi. (passing by about seven trail intersections!) As you near the Fairview entrance you should see an interesting rock garden. From there head south and again stay right. You will pass a tall graffitied concrete structure, cross a creek, and then pass another similar concrete structure whose original purpose eludes me. Perhaps they are the ruins of an ancient Roman aqueduct? At this point giving good directions becomes difficult due to the presence of several intersections of multiple trails of varying quality. From the second concrete tower, heading south and staying on larger trails will take you a section of trail paralleling the Promenade on Kavanaugh. After passing the two Promenade entrances, follow the trail to the right as it runs behind the church. Turn left onto the paved trail and head downhill for about 150 feet before turning right onto another dirt trail. If you are tired of rough trails at this point feel free to stay on the paved trail and follow it for half a mile back to your car. If you stay right on the dirt trail for about 1/3 of a mile, you will reach a grassy area near the baseball field. Head towards the playground and tennis court to return to your car or go explore some of the other trails in the park!

BOYLE PARK

Located between Col. Glenn. Rd., University Ave. and Kanis, with Rock Creek flowing through its center, Boyle Park is a large urban park with over 10 miles of both paved and unpaved trails. Many of these trails run along Rock Creek or side streams and ponds, providing access to fishing and good birding. The paved trails are well-maintained, fairly level, and excellent places for parents to take their small children or strollers. The dirt trails are typically much steeper and more rugged. They are used primarily by mountain bikers and hikers. If you visit the park be sure to notice the interesting clump of tupelo trees right at the car bridge across Rock Creek.

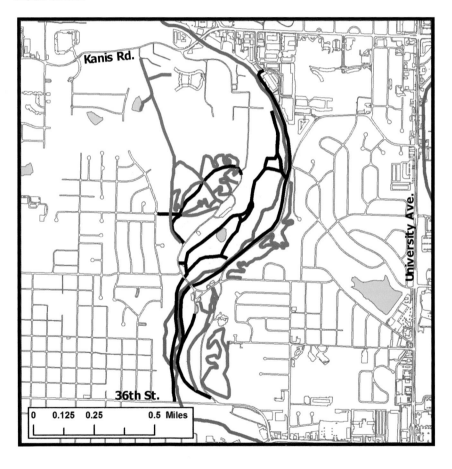

BOYLE PARK – EAST

Southern Ridge Trail

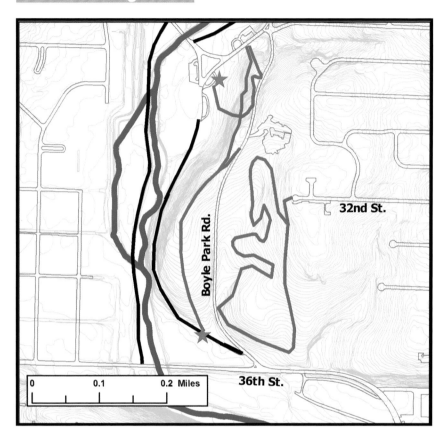

Start: 34°43′ 33.8″N 92°21′ 26.6″W

End: 34°43′ 16.0″N   92°21′ 28.2″W

Length: 0.4 miles – One-way   **Scenery:** ★★★★

Difficulty: Medium – Steep in places, some roots and rocks in trail

This trail provides a nice unpaved alternative to old Park Road, the paved bike/pedestrian trail it parallels. There are several entrances to this trail located on the ridge between Boyle Park Road and the paved bike trail along Rock Creek.

This trail begins at the entrance behind pavilion #2 and heads up a steep hill. Gaining over 30 feet in elevation over about 100 feet, the beginning of this trail is the hardest part and usually gets my heart pumping. The next quarter mile of the trail is fairly level and scenic as it passes through a wooded area offering occasional views of Rock Creek. The trail ends after a short downhill, where it intersects the paved trail near Boyle Park Road.

This trail is most often used (and maintained) by bikers, so be alert if you are traveling on foot!

To make this trail longer, catch the Nun Trail located across Boyle Park Rd. and described on the next page.

Nun Trail

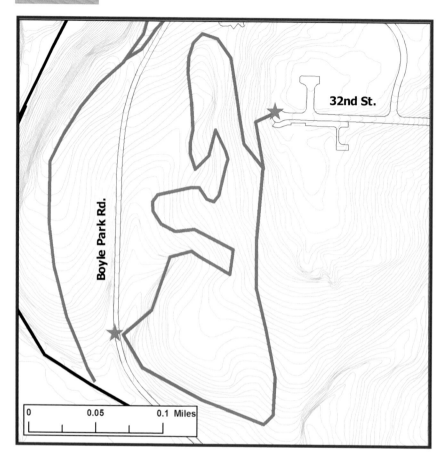

Trailheads:

Boyle Park Road: 34°43′17.14″N   92°21′26.76″W

32nd Street: 34°43′25.51″N   92°21′19.51″W

Length: 0.9 mile – Loop   **Scenery:** ★★★

Difficulty: Medium – Moderate elevation change and rocky

With entrances at Boyle Park Road and 32nd Street, this nearly one-mile loop winds its way through a forested area in the southeastern corner of Boyle Park. Used primarily by mountain bikers, the western half of the trail has several twists and turns. The eastern half is much straighter and runs along a fence for much of its length. It should be noted that I called this the Nun Trail due to the convent located near the 32nd St. trailhead, but my dad pointed out that the trail itself bears some resemblance to a praying nun.

Archwood Winding Trail

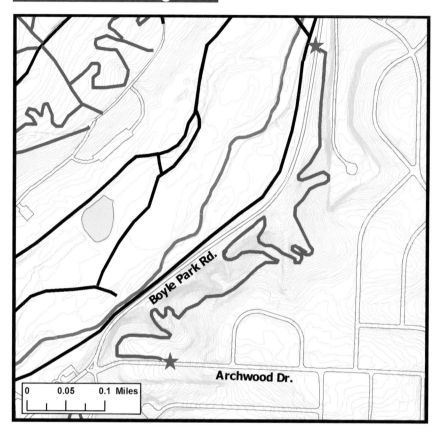

Start: 34°43' 38.6"N 92°21' 16.1"W

End: 34°43' 57.0"N   92°21' 01.8"W

Length: 0.9 miles – One-way   **Scenery:** ★★★⯪

Difficulty: Hard – Lots of elevation change and rocky

This extremely winding trail twists its way through an area bounded by Boyle Park Rd, Archwood Dr, and Broadmoor Neighborhood to the east of the park. Designed by mountain bikers, this trail doesn't get you anywhere quickly, but it really crams a fairly scenic hike into a small area in the middle of Little Rock. Paralleling about half a mile of Boyle Park Rd, it covers 0.9 miles. The trail starts at Archwood Dr, 0.1 miles east of Boyle Park Rd. It starts out heading west and slightly downhill. After 0.1 miles the trail turns and heads right back uphill. Get used to this because this trail has lots of 180 degree turns that send you up and downhill often within view of the section of trail you were on a minute ago. After about 1/4 mile and seven sharp turns, the trail straightens and flattens out long enough for you to get your breath back before doing yet another series of twists and turns with some altitude change. About 2/3 of the way through, the trail straightens out again and heads downhill. The final 1/5 mile parallels Boyle Park Rd. and is very flat.

BOYLE PARK – WEST

Boyle Park West Outer Trail

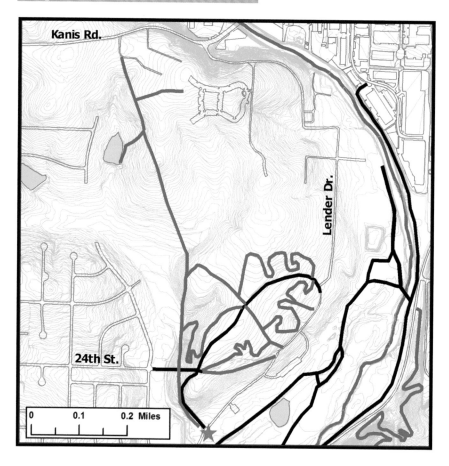

Start: 34°43'46.98"N 92°21'32.33"W

Length: 2.17 miles – Loop   **Scenery:** ★★★★

Difficulty: Medium – Some elevation change and rocky in places

Get on the dirt trail that begins in Boyle Park near where some large boulders block off an old paved road from the main road running through the western part of the park. Follow this fairly straight trail that runs along a gas pipeline right of way for 0.8 miles. Near Kanis short spurs lead to a small lake on one side and an apartment complex on the other. You might consider turning around at this point, since a fairly aggressive, unchained dog roams the trailer park where the trail hits Kanis. Heading back the way you came, take a left shortly after you re-cross the small stream. Follow this trail uphill for a tenth of a mile. Shortly before it hits the paved loop, the dirt trail forks. Take a sharp left and follow the dirt trail for 0.4 miles as it winds its way though the woods. At one point you will see a barbed wire fence. Shortly before you reach the fence you may see a less worn trail head off to the left, but be sure to stay right. The trail makes several sharp turns before straightening and intersecting the paved loop. Take a left on the paved trail and then a right when you hit the road. Follow the road for a third of a mile to get back to where you started or explore some of the numerous other trails in the vicinity.

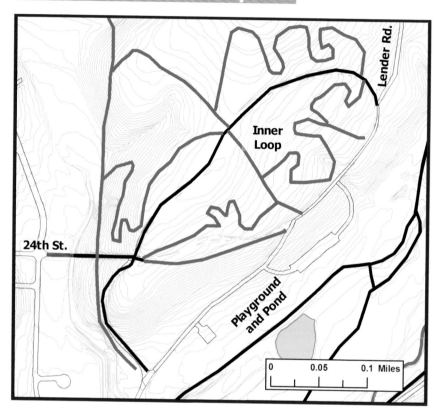

Trailheads:

1) 34°43′54.46″N 92°21′21.26″W   **3)** 34°43′58.63″N 92°21′26.09″W

2) 34°44′01.33″N 92°21′15.97″W   **4)** 34°43′52.68″N 92°21′31.54″W

Scenery: ★★★✦

Difficulty: Medium – slightly steep, rocky in places

This trail winds it way around the interior of the paved loop that is formed by an active road and a closed off road that is currently accessible only to bikers and pedestrians. This dirt trail can be accessed from many points around the paved loop and zig-zags around, cramming about ¾ miles of trail into a relatively small area.

BRODIE CREEK

Flowing from West Little Rock southeast until it joins Fourche Creek in Hindman Park, Brodie Creek is one of the most scenic creeks in town. This hidden gem doesn't have much in the way of developed trails, but for more adventurous readers these sites will amaze you with how far from civilization they make you feel while being surrounded by the city.

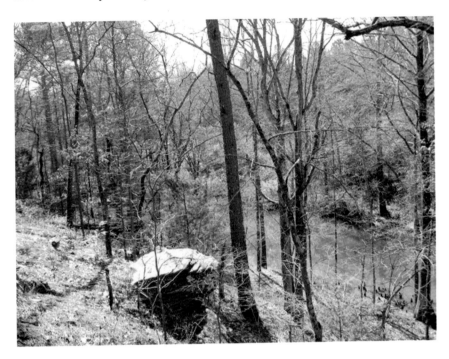

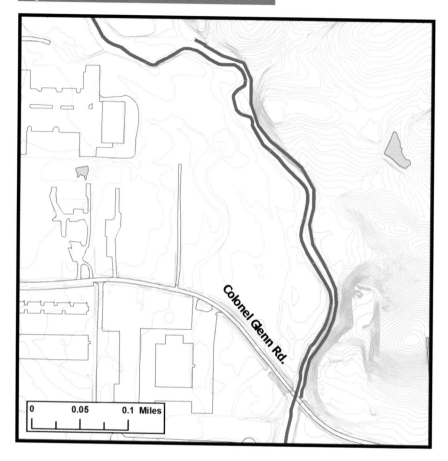

Start: 34°42′ 37.94″N 92°23′ 6.46″W

End: 34°42′ 53.10″N 92°23′ 9.45″W

Length: 0.3 miles – one-way   **Scenery:** ★★★★✦

Difficulty: Easy – fairly flat, but rough in places

This hike is one of my favorites in Little Rock. The scenery is outstanding. Large quartz infused boulders line mossy banks where large pines grow next to cypress trees. In the spring trout lilies, rue anemone, and other interesting flowers bloom along the trail. For much of the hike you have the clear waters of Brodie Creek flowing through cypress knees on one side and a steep forested hillside with rocky outcroppings on the other.

This trail begins on the north side of the Colonel Glenn bridge over Brodie Creek, just 0.4 miles west of the intersection with Stagecoach Rd. Parking on the street can be a bit scary so you might try parking at AIMCO about 200 yards west of the bridge.

Hiking along the right side of the creek, you will enter a beautiful forested area with a steep hillside on your right and Brodie Creek on your left. For the most part the trail is easy to follow, but in places it is overgrown. If you lose the trail your best bet is to just stay close to the creek until you find it again.

As you make your way along the creek, you'll pass several islands of varying sizes. Shortly after crossing a small ephemeral stream and passing a small island, you'll come across what is perhaps simultaneously the most scenic and unsightly part of the trail. An overturned bullet riddled car and several appliances mar a setting that you could otherwise confuse with being somewhere in Petit Jean State Park. The car lies on a steep hillside with a large rock overhang. Climbing this hill gives you a great view of the area. In the creek there is a big island lined with large river birch and pine.

A bit further up the creek you reach a point where a tributary and two branches of Brodie Creek come together. These can be hard to cross without getting wet, and just upstream the vegetation gets REALLY thick, making this a good point to turn around. If you aren't quite ready to turn around, feel free to turn to the right and explore the area around the smaller tributary.

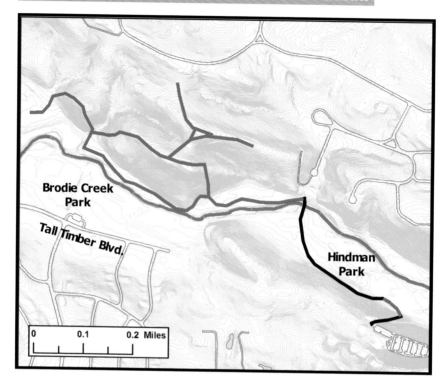

Start: 34°42′6.25″N 92°22′29.73″W

End: 34°42′4.70″N 92°22′8.17″W

Length: 0.35 miles – One-way   **Scenery:** ★★★✦

Difficulty: Medium – trail overgrown at times, steep side trails

Another section of Brodie Creek that is particularly scenic lies between aptly named Brodie Creek Park and Hindman Park. There is a dirt trail along the north side of the creek that is easy to follow in late fall and winter, but can be overgrown by the end of summer. For more exercise or to get away from the dense vegetation, there are some side trails that parallel this one along the hillside to the north. Steep trails lead to the upper trail in at least two places.

I like to park at Brodie Creek Park, located on Tall Timber Blvd. about 1/3 mile east of Stagecoach Rd., between Shackleford Rd. and Colonel Glenn. From the parking lot, head north to the creek. I typically cross near the eastern edge of the grassy area and pick up the dirt trail on the other side. Head east along the trail, keeping the creek on your right. In the spring you will encounter beautiful large patches of yellow and white trout lilies growing in this forested area of cypress, tupelo, oaks, and pines. After 1/3 mile, the trail reaches Hindman Golf Course. This makes a good turning around point if you are mostly interested in hiking more natural, forested locales; however the golf course can be quite scenic in its own right and is a good place to view wildlife. Great Blue Herons and beaver frequent the course's creeks and ponds, and spotted gar can be seen in Fourche Creek.

If the creek is too high to cross, you can follow the sewer right-of-way along the southern side of the creek, but this hike is much less scenic.

You can also avoid crossing Brodie Creek by hiking this route in reverse. Park at the golf club parking lot up on the hill in Hindman Park, walk out the west side of parking lot and follow the paved cart trail down hill for almost 100 yards. Turn left (north) and walk down the steep grassy hillside about 200 feet until you reach another cart trail. Turn left on the trail and follow it around the edge of the golf course for almost a third of a mile. Right after you cross Brodie Creek on the bridge, look to your left for a way into the woods. There are a few spots that all lead back to the trail, just make sure you find the trail that runs along the creek and heads west.

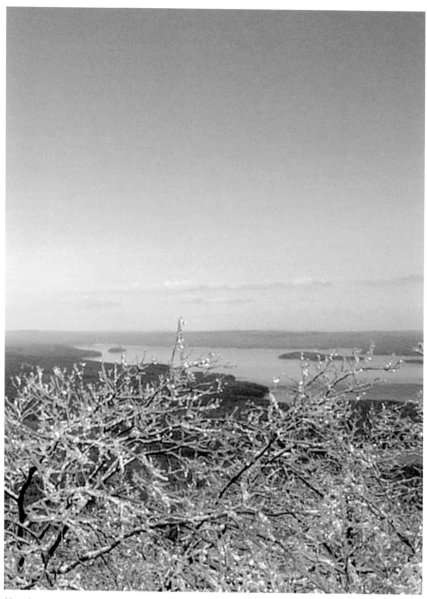

View from Pinnacle Mountain after an ice storm.

GILLAM PARK / AUDUBON NATURE CENTER

Gillam Park is the new home of the Audubon Arkansas Nature Center. This 400+ acre natural area is home to a wide variety of habitats including: a cypress oxbow, willow oak flats, bottomland hardwood forest, oak savanna, upland pine/white oak forest, and rare nepheline syenite glades. This book describes two trails at the center, but more are being built all the time, so look for more trails to be built in this park in the near future.

For more information on the trails or nature center (open Fall 2009), visit: ar.audubon.org or swing by the center located half a mile south of I-440 at the corner of Springer Blvd. and Gillam Park Rd.

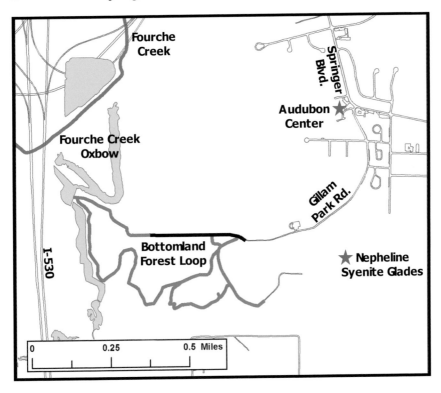

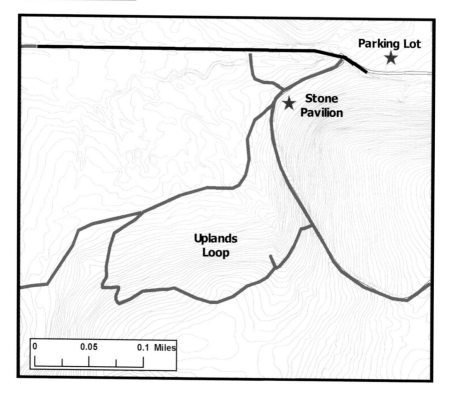

Start/End: 92°15′36.933″W 34°42′1.515″N

Length: 0.6 miles – Loop   **Scenery:** ★★★

Difficulty: Medium – moderate elevation change, rocky in places

This is a fairly new trail and is pretty rocky in places. Lots of muscadine, pine, white oaks, and poison ivy grow along the trail.

From the stone pavilion, head south (away from the parking lot) down the gravel road. Follow the gravel road past the metal gate and up the hill. After 0.14 miles, take a right onto the small trail branching off from the gravel road. If you reach a fence you've come too far.

About 100 yards after you leave the gravel road the trail will split. To the right is a short spur to a bench and wildlife watching area. The main trail heads uphill to the left for another hundred yards before leveling out. Over the next 0.2 miles you will head downhill over the newest and sometimes roughest part of the trail. At the bottom of the hill, the trail meets up with the Bottomland Forest and Oxbow Loop. Head right to get back to where you started or head left for a longer hike along the oxbow.

Bottomland Forest and Oxbow Loop

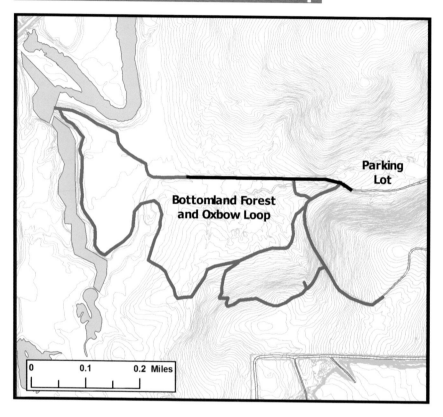

Start/End: 92°15′36.12″W 34°42′1.92″N

Length: 1.6 miles – Loop   **Scenery**: ★★★✦

Difficulty: Easy – flat, paved or gravel in places

Starting from the parking lot, head west past the metal gate and down the old paved road. Going counter-clockwise around this trail makes it easier to follow and takes you through the least scenic section first, thus saving the best for later. You will pass a gravel road heading off to your left and a dirt trail to the left just a little farther down the road.

After about 0.3 miles, the road switches from asphalt to gravel. The trail winds through a bottomland hardwood forest and along an oxbow of Fourche Creek for the next 0.75 miles. Along the way the gravel ends and gives way to a dirt trail. After walking along the edge of the cypress-lined lake for a while, the trail heads back into the woods. When you reach the power line right of way be sure to head straight and find the trail instead of getting on the power line right of way. The right of way heads towards the interstate to the right and to the paved part of this loop to the left.

The next third of a mile leads through a wooded area. The Uplands Loop Trail heads of to the right, but to get back to the parking lot quickly stay to the left and then turn left on the gravel road. You will pass a stone pavilion on your right before reaching the paved road you walked in on.

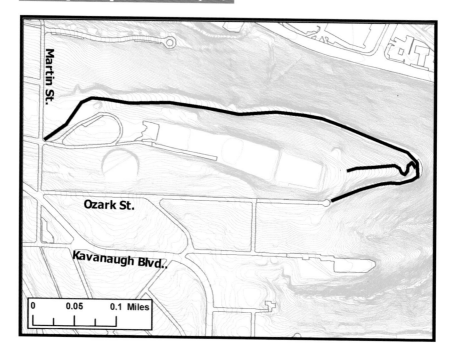

Start/End: 34°45′20.88″N   92°18′15.35″W

Length: 1.0 miles – Loop   Scenery: ★★★★

Difficulty: Easy – paved and flat

Knoop Park is tucked secretly away in Hillcrest and surrounds a water treatment plant. The trail through the park is paved and fairly flat, making for a short easy walk offering stunning views of Riverdale, Downtown, and the State Capitol. If you visit the park in the spring or early summer you may catch the wisteria in bloom. To get to Knoop Park, turn north off Kavanaugh onto Fairfax Terrace and then right onto Ozark Point. The road dead-ends at the entrance to Knoop Park.

From the parking area at the end of Ozark Point, head east along the trail. In about 0.1 miles you will reach the overlook area with nice benches and views of Downtown Little Rock, North Little Rock, and Riverdale. This spot is a great place to watch sunrise and 4th of July fireworks. A spur trail heads of to the left about 0.1 mi. up the hill and provides more views of downtown and the State Capitol.

From here the main trail heads west for about 1/2 mile through a wooded area that is home to the large patches of wisteria mentioned above. The trail has several benches and a water fountain and ends at Martin Street. At this point you could head back the way you came or do what I like to do and make it a loop by turning left on Martin and then left on Ozark. There are some unique houses along the way featuring interesting landscaping and architectural styles.

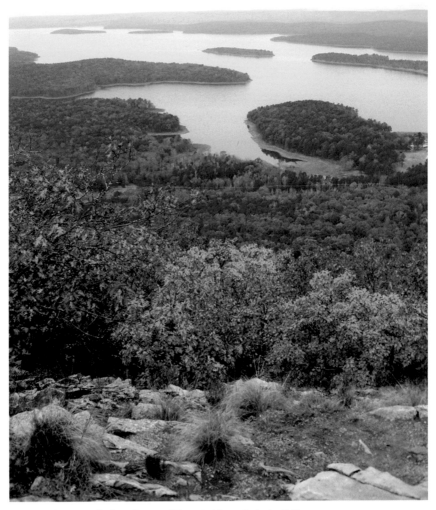

View of Lake Maumelle from the top of Pinnacle Mountain in the Fall.

PINNACLE MOUNTAIN

Pinnacle Mountain State Park is located near the Northwestern edge of Little Rock. The 70+ acre park has something for everyone: large fields, a playground, short paved trails through scenic bottomland forest, an arboretum, an educational visitor center, multiple put-ins on the Little Maumelle and Maumelle rivers, and several more rigorous hikes to the top of Pinnacle Mountain and other peaks in the area. The park maintains over 40 miles of paved, unpaved, and water trails. When you get to the park be sure to grab a copy of their trails brochure.

Since trails here are heavily trafficked, please stay on marked trails. Erosion is a major problem on the unpaved trails around the park and taking shortcuts or using old trails can make the problem worse.

More information on the park can be found at:
http://www.arkansasstateparks.com/pinnaclemountain

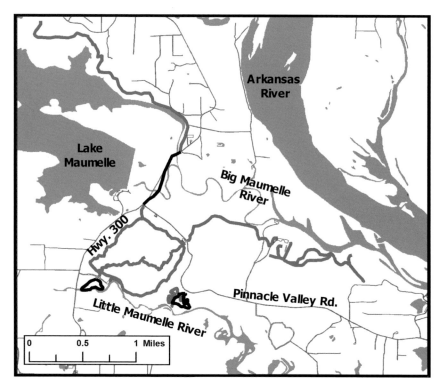

East Summit

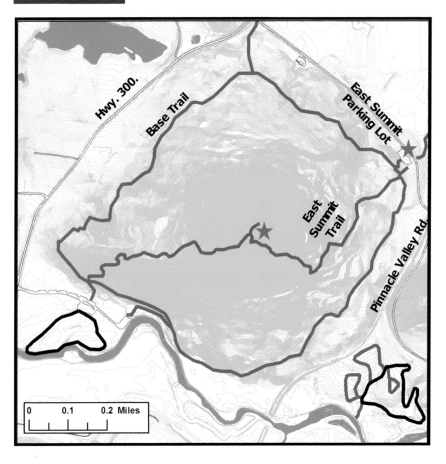

Start: 34°50′39.35″N   92°28′44.76″W

End: 34°50′29.12″N   92°29′9.13″W

Length: 0.75 miles – one-way   **Scenery**: ★★★★★

Difficulty: Very Hard – requires scrambling up steep boulder fields

This trail is the more difficult of the two trails leading to the top of Pinnacle Mountain and is perhaps the most rigorous trail in Little Rock. Parking for this trail is half a mile east of Hwy 300 on Pinnacle Valley Rd. Following the red and white blazes from the parking lot, the trail is initially lightly sloped and well worn. Both the East Summit and West Summit trails have markers numbered 1-10 to give you an idea of how far along the trail you are. The first six markers are deceptively easy to get to. After that point the trail becomes very steep and involves scrambling over large boulders. Watch where you put you feet since some rocks are slick and leaf covered gaps between boulders can hide ankle twisting holes! Since you will likely be stopping several times between markers 7 and 10, be sure to check out the amazing views along the way! If you have energy to burn, there are a couple large rock walls around markers 8 and 9 that are fun to climb around on. The trail ends at what I'll call "Peak 1" which offers good views of the Arkansas River, downtown Little Rock, and Chenal Mountain to the north, east, and south. A short rocky hike to the other peak gives you great views of Lake Maumelle off to the west as well. From the top you have the option of returning the way you came or going down the easier side and walking around the base of the mountain back to your car.

West Summit

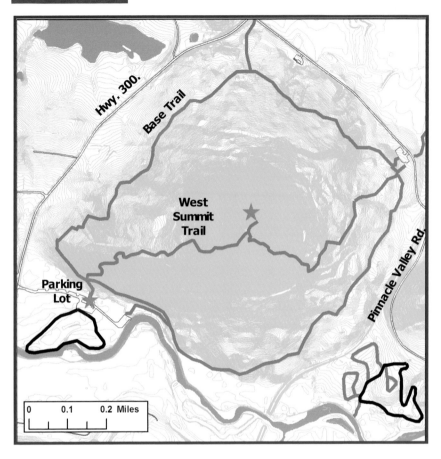

Start: 34°50′22.26″N 92°29′34.64″W

End: 34°50′31.63″N 92°29′7.62″W

Length: 0.78 miles – one-way   **Scenery**: ★★★★★

Difficulty: Hard

This is the easier of the two trails to the summit and by far the most popular. On a typical nice weekend the parking lot overflows and it isn't uncommon to pass dozens of people on your way to the top. If you prefer solitude try the East Summit trail, explore the other summits in the park, or go when it is really cold. I've gone up this side twice without encountering a single human being; once to see sunrise on New Years Day and the other immediately after a big ice storm.

This is a great trail to bring along the kids or dog.

The trail begins on the north side of the parking lot near the playground and restrooms. The well-worn and clearly marked trail heads gradually uphill for about 100 yards before you reach the intersection with the loop trail. Stay straight and follow signs for the West Summit Trail. About 200 yards later you will come to a short natural rock wall on your left. After almost half a mile, you will reach a large rock 'glacier' signaling that much of the rest of the trip to the top will involve hiking up large boulders. The trail is also much steeper from this point on up; luckily there are many great places to rest and take in some amazing views. As you near the top, the trail splits leading to the two different peaks. While both peaks provide near-360 degree views, the peak to the left offers better views to the north. The peak to the right has slightly better views of Little Rock and is where the East Summit trail ends.

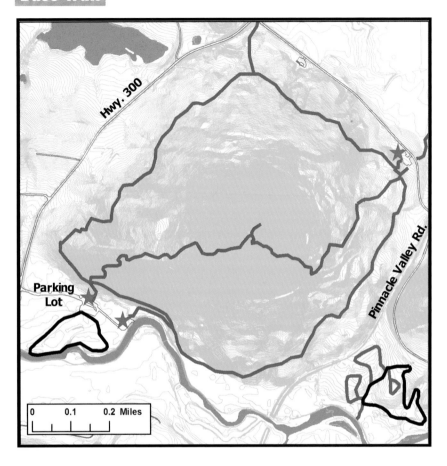

Trailheads:

West Summit Trail: 34°50′22.26″N   92°29′34.64″W

East Summit Trail: 34°50′39.35″N   92°28′44.76″W

West Side Canoe Launch: 34°50′19.80″N   92°29′28.64″W

Length: 3.0 miles – loop   **Scenery**: ★★★★

Difficulty: Medium

This trail connects the bases of the two summit trails making it possible to go up one side, down the other, and return to your car by walking around the base of the mountain. I enjoy going up the east side for more scrambling and fewer people and then down the west which is easier on the knees.

The Base Trail used to just run around the south side of the mountain, but a recently completed route around the northern side makes it possible to hike all the way around the mountain. Both sections are fairly scenic: the northern one winds through some rocky areas and past an old house while the southern route runs near the Little Maumelle for some distance. The northern route is the longer and more difficult of the two with a bit more elevation change, a rockier trail, and more switchbacks.

Kingfisher Trail

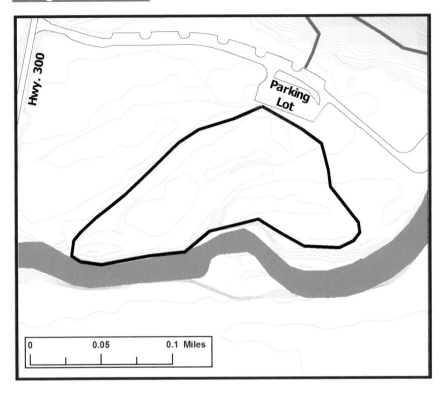

Start: 34°50'20.61"N   92°29'36.91"W

Length: 0.5 mi. – Loop   **Scenery:** ★★★★

Difficulty: Easy – short, flat, paved

Perhaps the least difficult of the trails in the park, the Kingfisher is a half mile, flat, handicapped accessible, paved trail with great views of the Little Maumelle. While the trails over and around the mountain are lined with hickories, oaks, and pines; this trail is home to sycamores, river birch, sweet gums, box elders, river cane, and enormous cypress trees. A huge hollowed out cypress tree with a face-sized hole in the trunk provides a great photo op for anyone who can squeeze into the opening in the back of the tree.

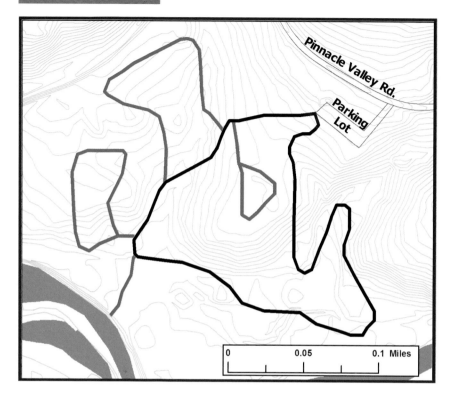

Start: 34°50′12.90″N 92°28′43.91″W

Length: 0.6 mi. – Loop   **Scenery:** ★★★✦

Difficulty: Easy – short, fairly flat, paved

The arboretum trail system consists of a 0.6 mile paved loop with several short dirt loop and spur trails connected to it. These trails are all fairly flat and there are plenty of benches along the way. Numerous informative signs line the trail providing information on our state's ecoregions and the species of trees found in each. Heading counter-clockwise around the trail, the 5th spur you reach will take you to a bench overlooking the Little Maumelle River.

Quarry Trail

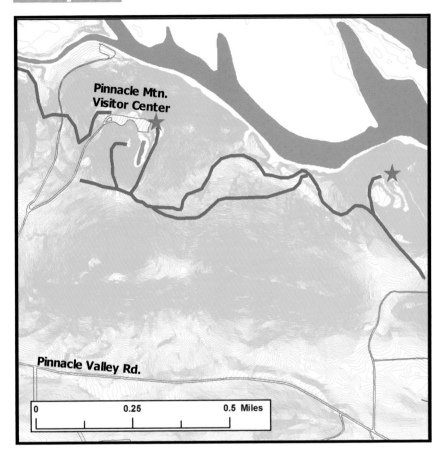

Start: 34°50′38.39″N 92°27′43.32″W

Length: 2.5 mi. – Round-Trip   **Scenery:** ★★★★

Difficulty: Medium – steep and rocky in places

The trail begins at the southeast corner of the Pinnacle Mountain Visitor Center parking lot near the quarry pond. The trail is paved for a short while before it turns left to an overlook over the Arkansas River. To follow the quarry trail, turn right onto the dirt trail. After 0.2 miles the quarry trail turns to the left. Staying straight on the road and then curving right up the hill will take you to an overlook of the quarry pond and the visitor center area.

After you turn left onto the Quarry Trail, go ~150 yards to where the trail forks. Take a left and head downhill. After about a third of a mile, the fairly rocky and eroded trail levels out into a smooth dirt trail and half a mile from the fork the two trails meet up again just past where a short spur trail leads down to the water for a view of the Maumelle River. Shortly after reaching this point, the trail heads uphill and becomes fairly steep. On your way up the hillside, look for an old car along the trail. After about a quarter mile of uphill you will reach an old road. The Quarry Trail follows the road to the left. If you follow the road to the right instead, you will pass a small quarry on the left and eventually exit the park on Norwood Road.

From the intersection with the old dirt road, the Quarry Trail continues for a few hundred yards to an open area with views of Pinnacle Mountain, an old quarry, the Arkansas River, the Maumelle River, and Lake Maumelle. When you are done exploring the area, head back the way you came. At the bottom of the hill turn left to take the other fork of the trail back. Shortly after crossing three bridges, you will meet up with the other fork of the trail. Head out the way you came in.

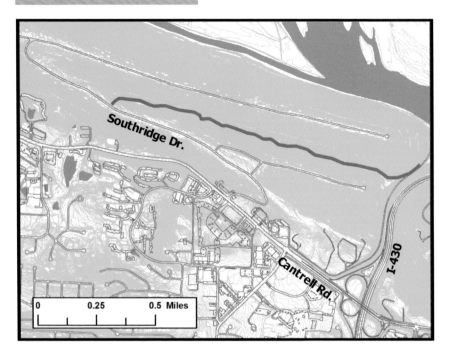

Start: 34°48′1.32″N 92°24′34.76″W – Off Southridge Dr.

End: 34°47′46.20″N 92°23′14.95″W – Off River Mountain Rd.

Length: 1.4 miles – one-way   **Scenery:** ★★★★✦

Difficulty: Medium – steep and rocky in places

This trail almost didn't appear in this book. I'd known of the park for a long time as it appears on city maps. I never heard anyone talk about it though, and figured it was just some land given to the city after developers had completed Walton Heights, to avoid paying extra taxes. There is still no marked entrance to this park and no official parking area nearby, but River Mountain Park hides a great secret. A very scenic and moderately difficult trail winds its way up the valley, crossing an amazingly beautiful creek many times. There are many interesting features of this creek, perhaps the most unique and stunning are where it flows in a perfectly straight line for hundreds of feet bounded on one bank by a high sheer rock wall.

You can park either along the River Mountain Road in a gravel pull-off area or further away at the parking lot on the Arkansas River where people put in boats or hit the River Trail. The trail is harder to find from this entrance but starts with the uphill, leaving you with the option to turn around an head downhill whenever you get tired.

However, the trail is easier to find at its upstream entrance where a powerline crosses Southridge in the Walton Heights neighborhood. Park at the crossing and head north along the power line right-of-way. Turn right just past the end of the fence and keep your eyes peeled for small white rectangles nailed to trees which mark most of this trail. The trail heads down through a beautiful valley paralleling a small stream. The spring is a great time to hike this trail, since it is home to numerous dogwoods. The rocky valley slopes are covered in pines, white oaks, and ironwood trees among others. If you explore off trail, higher up on the slopes you can find some Blackjack oaks as well. In many places the trail is lined with ferns and mayapples. The trail crosses the creek in numerous places and can be fairly rough and hard to follow at times. As you near River Mountain Road (at about the 1.2 mile mark), the trail blazes end and you can either turn around and follow them back up to your car or continue heading east finding your own path to the road.

RIVER TRAIL

The River Trail is a paved bike/pedestrian trail that runs along both the North Little Rock and Little Rock sides of the Arkansas River. Parking for the trail can be found at numerous locations along the trail including:

1) Under I-430 on River Mountain Rd.

2) Burns Park in North Little Rock

3) Murray Park

4) Rebsamen Park

River Trail Loop from River Mountain Road

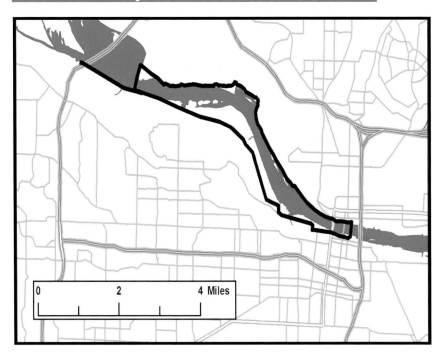

Start/End: 34°47'43.61"N   92°22'38.45"W

Length: 16.25 miles – Loop   **Scenery:** ★★★★✦

Difficulty: Easy – paved and flat

To reach the parking lot at River Mountain Road, take Cantrell west, and turn right on River Mountain Road, at its intersection with Cantrell and Old Rodney Parham Road. Follow the road for about 1.5 miles, under I-430 to where it dead ends at the River Trail. Take the trail east for about 1 mile and then get on the recently completed Big Dam Bridge. Getting to the top of the bridge is probably the hardest part of this trail. Once you get to the top it is *mostly* flat and downhill from here. Take a break on the bridge and look west to see Two Rivers Park, the Little Maumelle, and Pinnacle Mountain. Sunsets from the bridge can be quite amazing. To the east you can see Rebsamen Park, Burns Park, and the cliffs of Emerald Park. When you come down on the North Little Rock side of the bridge you enter the most scenic section of the trail. The next 4 miles takes you through wooded areas, across Burns Park, and into Emerald Park. There are lots of side trails in Emerald Park that take you to the foot of the beautiful 200 ft. cliffs or even up to the top if you've got energy to spare. The views of downtown Little Rock from the top of Emerald Park are quite impressive.

From here the trail heads into downtown North Little Rock and through their riverfront park. Bicyclists and pedestrians currently cross into Little Rock on the recently opened Junction Bridge. You can also cross on the Main St. Bridge.

Once in Little Rock, the trail follows city roads for quite a while. If you have extra time and energy, take a detour and head east on the trail along the river to see the Farmer's Market, the Medical Mile, the new Arkansas Game and Fish center, and Clinton Library.

The trail roughly follows Cantrell Rd, to Riverfront Dr., before becoming a real bike/pedestrian trail once again at the intersection of Rebsamen Road and Riverfront Dr. On your right you'll see Rebsamen Golf Course and then Murray Park before reaching the Big Dam Bridge once again and continuing on to the parking lot. The exact route of the trail in the Downtown Little Rock area is subject to change so be on the lookout for signs.

More information can be found at: http://www.rivertrail.org

Rock Creek Trail

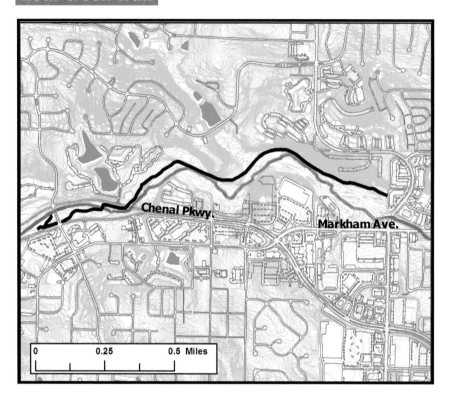

Start: 34°45′16.52″N 92°25′38.90″W

End: 34°45′19.50″N 92°24′25.19″W

Length: 1.4 miles – One-way   **Scenery:** ★★★✦

Difficulty: Easy – paved and flat

Though there are many sections of trail along Rock Creek, that will hopefully one day all be connected, the section I'm calling "Rock Creek Trail" refers solely to the relatively new paved trail in West Little Rock that runs between Loyola Dr. and Bowman Rd. For information on other sections of the trail along Rock Creek go to the Boyle Park trails section of this book.

This trail begins at the southern intersection of Loyola Dr. and Chenal Pkwy. You can park at the gas station or along the shoulder on Chenal if you are brave! The other entrance is located behind the shopping center at Bowman and Markham Place Dr. which has plenty of parking.

Starting from Loyola, the trail heads into the woods and parallels Rock Creek. Much of this section of the creek has been heavily "maintained" by the city and isn't too scenic. However, once you pass under Chenal Parkway you will enter a more natural section of the trail where things have been less disturbed. There are several great views of the creek along this part of the trail and be on the lookout for beautiful tupelo stands.

TWO RIVERS PARK

Two Rivers Park in West Little Rock, is one of the city's newest parks. With miles of paved, gravel, and grassy trails as well as a canoe launch providing easy access to the Little Maumelle and Arkansas Rivers, Two Rivers Park has something for everyone from toddlers tricycling on one of the flat paved trails to kayakers looking for a long all day paddle to Pinnacle Mountain and back. In a addition to the trail described on the next page, there is a network of easy flat trails, some paved, some gravel, in the southern portion of the park. At the time of writing, a bike/pedestrian bridge over the Little Maumelle was being discussed which would connect the park's trails to the River Trail.

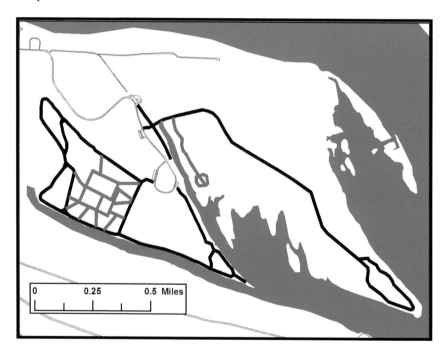

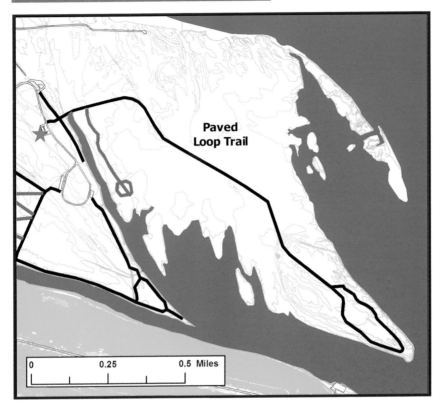

Start/End: 34°48′41.44″N   92°24′6.31″W

Length: 3.0 miles – Loop   **Scenery:** ★★★★

Difficulty: Easy – paved and flat

This flat paved semi-loop trail is great for a short jog or easy bike ride. It offers interesting views of a variety of habitats including swamp, bottomland hardwood forest, grassland, and pine forest. The trail begins across the road from the 2nd parking lot on your right about _miles into the park. You will briefly pass through a swampy section before the trail opens up into a large grassy area where it is not uncommon to spot large numbers of deer. A short grassy side trail leads off to your right.

As you continue down the paved trail, you will encounter more wetland areas with lots of horsetail growing along the trail. After about 1.2 miles, the trail splits to form a short loop. To the left you will enter a dense pine stand. To the right there is an open grassy area.

At the far end of the trail treat yourself to some great views of the Arkansas River and the I-430 bridge. There are picnic tables for anyone who feels like carrying supplies this far.

Water Trails

In addition to having a wide selection of trails for hiking and biking in our city, Little Rock is also home to several great water trails. With the Arkansas River on its northern edge, the Maumelle and Little Maumelle to the west, and Fourche Creek flowing through the city from the Otter Creek area in the southwest, to the airport on the eastern edge of town; Little Rock is surrounded with floating opportunities. No matter where in the city you live, you are within a few miles of a put-in.

FOURCHE CREEK

Fourche Creek is the least floated of the options mentioned above, though it is perhaps the most conveniently located. It flows past numerous public parks including: Otter Creek Park, Hindman Park, Benny Craig, Fourche Bottoms, Interstate Park, and Remmel Park. There are developed launches at Benny Craig Park, Interstate Park, and Remmel Park, but it is fairly easy to launch from Hindman too. At the time of this writing, a new launch was planned for a borrow pond under the interchange of Interstates 440, 530, and 30. An access road off of Arch St. just south of Interstate Park will take you to the pond, which has a small cypress knee lined connection to Fourche Creek.

Though it is relatively short, Fourche Creek flows through three of Arkansas' six major ecoregions. Over a day-long float the scenery changes from a gravel-bottom stream lined with river birch, box elder, and sycamore to a highly sinuous silt-bottomed creek lined with enormous cypress and silver maples.

This unique creek gives paddlers a taste of scenic wilderness while providing frequent reminders that you are actually in the state's most populous city.

Much more information on the creek can be found at:
http://www.fourchecreek.org

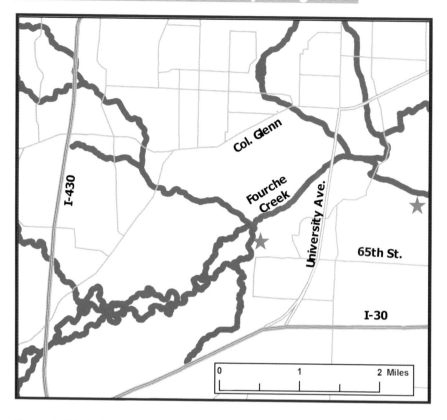

Start: 34°41'46.38"N   92°21'39.23"W (Hindman Park)

Finish: 34°42'10.09"N   92°19'36.60"W (Benny Craig Park)

Length: 2.4 mi. – One way   **Scenery:** ★★★✦

Difficulty: Medium – depending on flow you might have to portage frequently

Though this section is labeled as starting at I-430, this description begins with putting in at Hindman Park. Launching near I-430 either at the Highway Department or across the creek at the nursery can be tricky, but is definitely worth it. That section of the creek is quite scenic and completely devoid of other people. Of note for plant people, the banks of Fourche Creek in this area are home to the very rare Arkansas Meadow-rue.

A much easier place to put-in in this section is Hindman Park. If you want to float upstream on Fourche it is best to park on the gravel shoulder near the southern entrance to the park and put-in near the rock vane that has been constructed in the creek. If you are looking to float down to Benny Craig, you might want to put in a little further downstream at the bridge.

From the bridge paddle downstream past the north end of the golf course. Spotted gar and green herons are pretty common in this area. After about a quarter mile, the creek leaves the power line right of way and enters a forested stretch. There is often a several foot high beaver dam around this point that can be ramped over, or for the less adventurous, portaged around. The creek is fairly straight and scenic for the next ¾ of a mile. Look for some large cypress with dozens of knees! Of possible side interest to geology buffs, one of the easternmost outcroppings of novaculite (found in the Ouachita Mountains) can be found along the steep hillside to your right.

At the 1.0 mile mark, the creek enters an unsightly stretch where it has been channelized and dredged for flood control and to protect University Ave. When passing under the bridge, be on the lookout for swallows, which can put on quite a show for intruders at certain times of the year. After about half a mile, Rock Creek, the largest tributary of Fourche, pours into the creek on the left. The creek then heads into the woods again. After ~0.1 miles, Fourche Creek forks. Take the channel to the right, which is usually the only branch with much water in it anyways. Be sure you take the correct route since these forks of the creek don't come back together over 6 miles!

As the creek gradually turns to the right, you might see a man-made pond just over the bank to your right. The creek connects to this pond, but I don't recommend making a side trip into it. Just past the 2-mile mark, you pass under Mabelvale Pike. Just past the bridge you may have to portage around a yellow trash boom. From here, the canoe launch at Benny Craig park is a short straight 0.6 mi. trip with BFI landfill on your left and the launch coming up on your right. If you pass under a railroad bridge you've gone about a quarter-mile too far! Benny Craig Park is located near the intersection of Gum Springs Rd. and Rosemoor Dr.

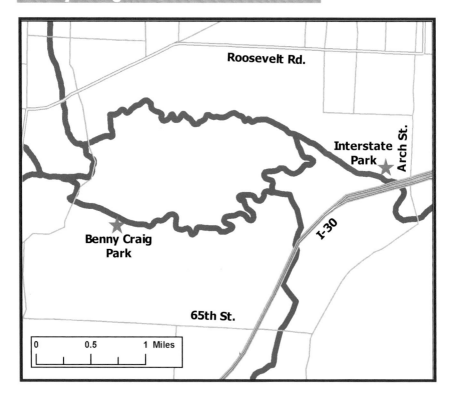

Start: 34°42′10.09″N   92°19′36.60″W

Finish: 34°42′29.05″N   92°17′6.36″W

Length: 4.4 mi. – One way   **Scenery**: ★★★★↵

Difficulty: Medium – depending on flow you might have to portage frequently

Easily the most frequently floated section of Fourche Creek, the middle section is where great scenery and ideal water depth overlap. Official concrete put-ins can be found at Benny Craig Park and Interstate Park. Unlike many popular floating destinations around the state, the 1.5 mile stretch of Fourche Creek upstream of Interstate Park is floatable year-round with no scrapping or portaging. A highly recommended and more detailed map of this section can be found at: http://www.fourchecreek.org/Floating.html

The launch at Benny Craig Park, located near the intersection of Gum Springs Rd. and Rosemoor Dr., is a very short walk north from the parking lot. Follow the creek to your right to head downstream, where just past the park you will pass under an active railroad bridge. A few minutes later you will reach an elevated gas pipeline that you may have to portage around. After 0.75 miles, you will come to a sharp bend in the creek with concrete all over the right bank. During low flow be careful not to scrape your boat on the concrete.

Shortly after you pass the concrete banks, you will come upon an elevated sewer line. Since all the landmarks I've mentioned so far might sound ugly, I feel compelled to mention that this section of the creek is actually quite scenic with cypress, silver maples, and box elder lining the banks. That said, due to the creek's size and sinuosity, unsightly trash tends to pile up in large mats at multiple locations along this stretch of the creek. This is a problem that Audubon Arkansas and the City of Little Rock are working on, but one that will likely take decades to solve.

After 2.2 miles you will come to the first of three large power line crossings. At the 3 mile mark, the creek begins to widen after you pass by the third large power line crossing. After a couple large bends, the creek becomes wider and fairly straight and deep for the last 1 mile leg to Interstate Park. The one exception, involves a difficult to spot sharp left turn you will need to make about 0.6 miles upstream of the takeout at 34°42′39.62″N 92°17′38.34″W. Hopefully this spot will be marked with an "Arkansas Water Trails" sign by the time this book is in print. However, if you happen to find yourself at a dead end, you've passed the turn and need to backtrack about 100 yards and look for your turn. If you hate backtracking you can always just portage 40 to 50 yards to the east and meet back up with the creek.

From here it is a short, easy float to Interstate Park. You'll know you are getting close when you reach the wooden railroad bridge. To give you some idea of how high flood waters can get here, I've seen a large dead tree stuck about 9 feet up on the bridge! About 120 yards past the bridge is the takeout at the southern edge of Interstate Park.

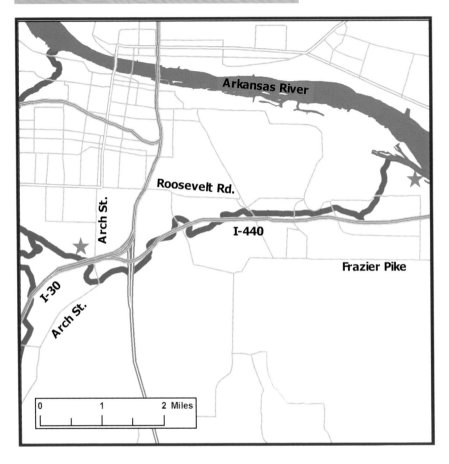

Start: 34°42′29.05″N   92°17′6.36″W

Finish: 34°43′34.72″N   92°11′16.51″W

Length: 7.6 mi. – One way   **Scenery**: ★★★✦

Difficulty: Medium – depending on flow you might have to portage some.

This float begins at Interstate Park and heads downstream. This is an interesting float but overall, not the most classically scenic. Since much of the route is wide and deep, this section can be much busier than areas upstream. Be ready to share the creek with motorboats and jet skis. Interstate 440 and the airport are never far away, making this the noisiest section of the creek to float.

Immediately after leaving the canoe launch, you will pass under a power line and then under Interstate 30. The next 0.7 miles are the most scenic of the float. The creek is narrow and surrounded by cypress. A short distance from the creek explorers can find numerous beaver dams on small side streams and large cypress trees with seven foot knees!

After passing under Arch Street, the creek immediately widens. Although not easily seen from the water, there is an old home foundation on the north side of the creek in this section. About half a mile past the bridge, a small cypress knee lined channel connects the creek to a large borrow pond that will have a canoe launch accessible from Arch St. starting sometime in 2009.

Less then 0.1 miles past the entrance to the borrow pond, the creek passes under Interstate 530. The next 0.4 miles are perfectly straight where the railroad cuts off a stretch of the original channel of Fourche Creek forming an oxbow lake that is part of the Audubon Arkansas Nature Center. If you pay close attention, you can find where the oxbow drains under the railroad. A rough portage under the railroad and over a large beaver dam will provide you with a nice side-float on the scenic lake.

Continuing on the main (straightened) channel of the creek you will pass by a large borrow pond to the north and then under I-440 several times over the next 0.75 miles.

At the 2.7 mi. mark, the trail passes under Springer Blvd. and loses most of its natural character for the rest its path to the Arkansas River. Just before you pass under Springer and bid farewell to scenic tree-lined sections of the creek, look for an odd cylindrical brick structure on the north side of the creek. Feel free to e-mail me if you have some good guesses as to what it was used for.

During the first half-mile downstream of Springer Blvd. you will pass under multiple highway on-ramps and off-ramps and I-440. The drastically altered channel then widens to about 150 feet. Over the next 2.75 miles, the creek passes under I-440, a railroad bridge, Airport Road, and Lindsey Road before reaching the boat launch at Remmel Park (34°43′0.69″N 92°12′23.71″W). This makes a good put-in or take out spot as there are no developed launches further downstream. Half a mile downstream of Remmel Park, you will reach the last place where it might be feasible to take-out or put-in, at Fourche Dam Pike. Along this road, near the creek, there is a Civil War plaque, marking the Engagement at Fourche Bayou that occurred on September 10th 1863. It'd be great to see a photograph from this battle, since I'm sure the creek must have looked very different from its current widened, mowed, and rip-rapped state.

From Fourche Dam Pike it is just over a mile to the creek's confluence with the Arkansas River.

LITTLE MAUMELLE

The Little Maumelle is generally regarded as the most scenic float in Little Rock. Over 8 miles of floatable creek offer stunning views of Pinnacle Mountain, dense groves of cypress, cattail stands and the I-430 Bridge. Canoes can be rented at the Pinnacle Mountain Visitor Center.

There are numerous places to put-in along the Little Maumelle including:

- Pinnacle Mtn. Canoe Launch at east end of parking lot –
  34°50′19.08″N 92°29′28.14″W

- House on Burnett Road off Pinnacle Valley Road (pay ~$5)
  34°48′53.54″N 92°26′26.03″W

- Bait Store off River Valley Marina Rd. Near Two Rivers –
  34°48′45.48″N 92°25′7.72″W

- Two Rivers Park – 34°48′28.71″N 92°23′55.59″W

- Boat Launch/River Trail Access Off River Mountain Rd. –
  34°47′55.63″N 92°23′7.06″W

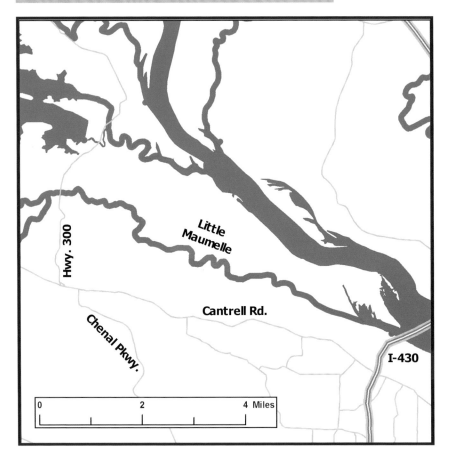

Start: 34°50′19.08″N   92°29′28.14″W

End: 34°48′28.71″N   92°23′55.59″W

Length: 9.0 miles – one-way   **Scenery:** ★★★★★

Starting at the boat launch at the far end of the West Summit parking lot, head downstream (to the left facing the creek). For the first few minutes the creek parallels a branch of the base trail, so be on the lookout for hikers to wave at. After a quarter mile or so the stream narrows and turn to the left, passing through some cypress knee rapids. If the water is low, you may have to get out and pull you boat through this section. Be sure to keep an eye out for turtles and snakes sunning themselves on trees and logs in the middle of the water. A railroad bridge marks the half-mile point and makes a good turn around point if you are looking for a short float. There isn't usually much of current in the Little Maumelle, so be sure to give yourself plenty of time if you plan to do all nine miles!

Continuing down the trail, you will pass under a high voltage power line. About a mile later, the creek opens up and becomes a bit harder to follow. Several side streams, islands, thick cypress stands and deceiving dead ends make exploring this area a fun but time-consuming task. To stay on track be sure to bring a good map (either in this book, on Google earth, or elsewhere). This trail may soon (or already) be marked with Arkansas Water Trail blazes, making navigation much easier. One of my favorite parts of the trail is located just past the two mile mark. Where a dense grove of cypress stands in the channel. Quietly weaving your way through this half-mile section of trail, you can surprise ducks, herons, turtles, snakes, and fishermen in flat-bottom boats. At the 3.5 mile mark, the trail passes under 2 large pipes and then enters three large bends with large islands. Much of the year one side of the islands is impassable due to shallow water and large amounts of vegetation, but those paths less traveled can provide a fun, challenging shortcut under the right conditions. Shortly after you pass under Pinnacle Vally Road, you will see a powerline crossing the creek. At the time this was written, you could pay five dollars to park and put-in or take out at this house located at the end of Burnett Road. Some of the land here has been up for sale, so putting in here may not be an option much longer.

Another fun place to take-out or at least take a break is the bait shop near Two Rivers Park, located at about the 6 mile mark. Park the kayaks and grab a soda and some snacks from this unique store before embarking on the final leg of the float. For the next 1.5 miles, Two Rivers Park is to your left and a railroad and Walton Heights neighborhood are to your right. When the trail opens up you have the choice of either hanging a sharp left and traveling half a mile to the canoe launch at Two Rivers Park or staying straight, heading towards the I-430 bridge, and taking out at the boat launch located off of River Mountain Road. This parking lot can be used to access the River Trail or River Mountain Trail.

The trail is dominated by cypress, but large silver maple, sycamores, river birch, water oaks, and shagbark hickory are also found along the banks. In the Spring and Summer you will probably see turtles and snakes sunning themselves. Deer occasionally swim across the Little Maumelle. In the summer large blooming lily pads cover huge swathes of the creek.

Potential/Upcoming Trails

This section of the book contains information on trails being planned or worked on.

If you would like to see more trails built in the city (including the ones on the pages that follow) there are several steps you could take:

1. Contact the mayor and city board of directors and let them know that you appreciate our parks and trails and would like to see more. Mention that you support the Open Space Policy Initiative described in detail at:
   http://www.littlerock.org/ParksRecreation/blog/

2. Contact the County Judge and let him know you appreciate the county's work on trails and would like to see more built.

3. Contact your state and federal representatives to let them know you support funding for parks and trails projects. There are often projects that have already been approved but that funding hasn't been appropriated for. One example of this is the approved, but so far unfunded, Corps of Engineers project in Fourche Bottoms. If funded completely, this project would include the construction of an access road, boardwalks, and canoe launch in the ~2,000 Fourche Bottoms area in the center of Little Rock.

Coleman Creek Greenway Trail

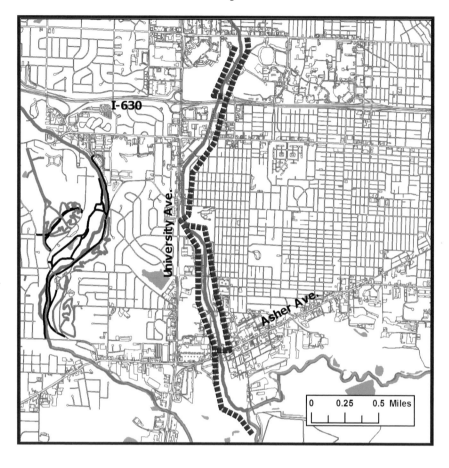

Spanning approximately 3 miles from Markham St. near War Memorial Stadium south to Fourche Creek near Asher Ave. and University Ave., this trail will follow Coleman Creek through War Memorial Park and the UALR Campus. The different sections of this trail are at various levels of the planning process. You can already see the beginnings of the trail at the southern end of UALR and within ten years there will be a paved trail running along both sides of the creek for the entire length of campus.

The creek and trails in War Memorial Park are undergoing improvements and expansion and will likely be completed in a few years.

Connecting these two sections initially will likely involve placing bike lanes and sidewalks along existing roads, with the hope of placing a bike and pedestrian only trail closer to the creek at a later date.

Completion of the southernmost section of this trail from Asher Ave. to Fourche Creek will depend on who comes to own the old Coleman Dairy Property and what they decide to do with it.

Rose Creek Trail

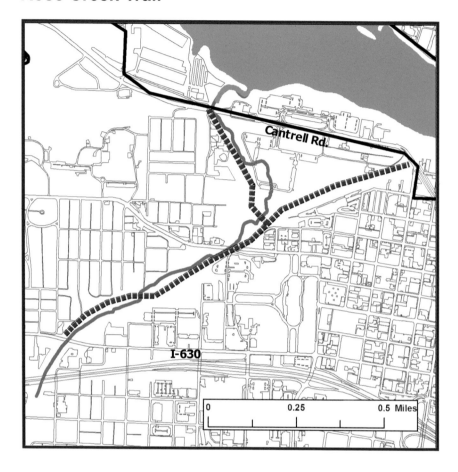

A trail along Rose Creek in the Capitol View, Stift Station neighborhoods was considered and partially planned many years ago. A renewed interest by the neighborhoods and city government in connecting the River Trail to these neighborhoods and perhaps all the way to 7th St. or Interstate 630 means this trail could one day become a reality. This trail could be used by people commuting by bike or foot from these areas to downtown.

Audubon Nature Center / Gillam Park

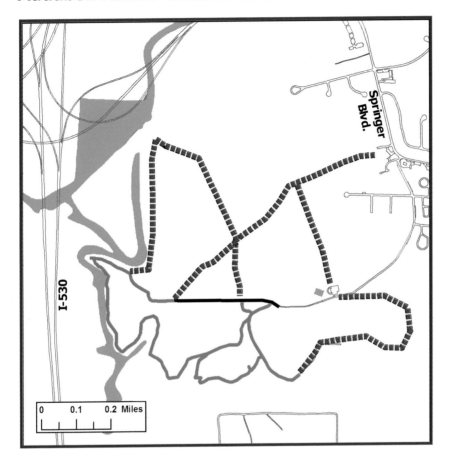

Though two trails at the Nature Center are included in this book, there are many more planned for the park. A trail will eventually run from behind the Nature Center building on Springer Blvd. up the grassy hill and through the woods to connect with the other trails in the park. Other trails there will link to rare nepheline syenite glades that are home to cacti and other unique plants. A canoe launch will be built to improve floating access to the Fourche Creek oxbow lake on the property.

Two Rivers Park

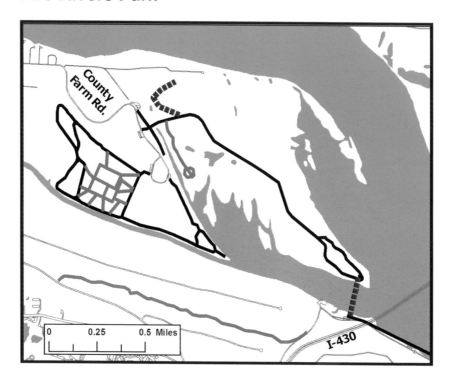

There are also more trails in the works for Two Rivers Park. Another unpaved trail will soon branch off from the 3-mile paved loop trail to the north. There may also soon be a bike and pedestrian bridge over the Little Maumelle River connecting the River Trail to the trails at Two Rivers. The plan is to eventually provide a way for people to bike from downtown Little Rock all the way to Pinnacle Mountain State Park where they would then have access to great floating opportunities on two creeks and hiking on numerous trails including the 223 mile Ouachita Trail.